AB WHEEL
WORKOUTS

AB WHEEL

WORKOUTS

Dr. Karl Knopf

50 Exercises to Stretch and Strengthen Your Abs, Core, Arms, Back and Legs

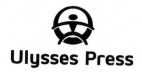

Ulysses Press

Published in the United States by
Ulysses Press
P.O. Box 3440
Berkeley, CA 94703
www.ulyssespress.com

ISBN: 978-1-61243-233-5
Library of Congress Control Number 2013938278

Printed in the United States by United Graphics Inc.

10 9 8 7 6 5 4 3 2 1

Acquisitions: Katherine Furman
Managing editor: Claire Chun
Editor: Lily Chou
Proofreader: Elyce Berrigan-Dunlop
Indexer: Sayre Van Young
Cover design: what!design @ whatweb.com
Photographs: © Rapt Productions except page 9 ab wheel © Lasse Kristensen/
    shutterstock.com; page 12 muscle anatomy © Sebastian Kaulitzki/shutterstock
    .com; page 14 skeleton © leonello calvetti/shutterstock.com
Models: Bryan Johnson, Lache Kamani

Distributed by Publishers Group West

Please Note
This book has been written and published strictly for informational purposes, and in no way should be used as a substitute for actual instruction with qualified professionals. The author and publisher are providing you with information in this work so that you can have the knowledge and can choose, at your own risk, to act on that knowledge. The author and publisher also urge all readers to be aware of their health status and to consult health care professionals before beginning any health program.

contents

PART 1

overview

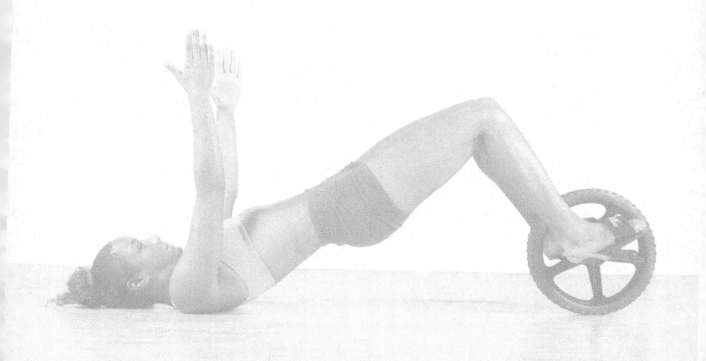

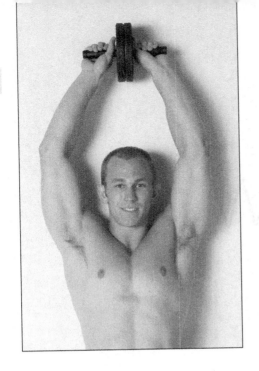

introduction

Looking for a unique approach to tone up your midsection, butt and back muscles? Look no further than the abdominal wheel! The "wheel" was extremely popular in the 1960s and was first advertised as a tool strictly for abdominal exercise. It lost some of its appeal because people were not using it properly and thought all you needed to melt away your belly fat was five minutes of ab wheel exercises. Of course, they were wrong.

When the ab wheel is used properly, however, it offers a fun and effective way to challenge your core stability as well as tone your upper and lower bodies. Most ab wheel exercise manuals show you how to do a few basic exercises, with the only modifications being to go left and right instead of straight ahead. I'm old enough to have used an ab wheel 50 years ago in my training, and I remember why the ab wheel waned in popularity: because it was boring and one-dimensional! My goal with *Ab Wheel Workouts* was to think outside the box to make training with the ab wheel more interesting.

Ab Wheel Workouts strives to provide total core training, incorporating old-school exercise approaches, Pilates and yoga. It also includes some flexibility exercises. With the comprehensive ab wheel training routine set forth in this book you can focus on your upper abs and lower abs as well as the "love handle" area. Soon you'll be on your way to better posture, a stronger core, and a fitter body.

what is an ab wheel?

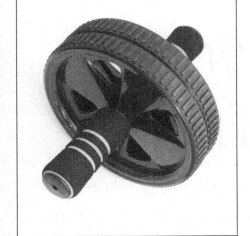

The ab wheel is a device that has a wheel with handles protruding from either side of it, allowing you to place your hands on either side of the wheel. While most ab wheels have a single wheel, you can also find some with two wheels, which offer better balance. The design is simple but the results can be fantastic if done in concert with sensible eating and adequate aerobic exercise.

The basic single- or dual-wheel ab wheel with handles is an inexpensive way to find out if you enjoy this type of training. These are so popular that they can be purchased at major drugstores, sporting goods stores and even discount stores for under $10. One advantage is that they're portable—they can be disassembled to fit in a small box or briefcase.

Some ab wheels feature a foot strap, which adds versatility but is not necessary; in most cases, an exercise band wrapped around the foot and handle provides the same support.

The elaborate versions, which have a spring recoil device that makes returning to the starting position much easier, are bigger and more costly. These are recommended for folks who have a hard time maintaining neutral spine position. However, note that you should not perform ab wheel training if you have lower back issues, poor spinal stability, upper body weakness or even high blood pressure.

The bottom line is: Whichever version you select can produce the same results. Remember, the end result is dependent on variables such as time on task, aerobic exercise and avoiding excessive calories. All the exercises in this book can be done with the $10 or $50 version, the choice is yours. The more expensive version will not give you any better results. In fact, no piece of equipment can do it for you—it takes effort.

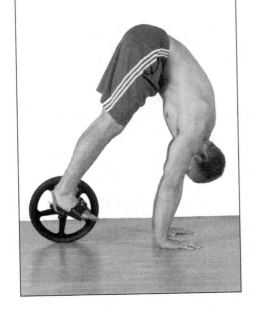

benefits of ab wheel training

The ab wheel is just another tool in the fitness toolbox that targets your core, and it does so by challenging your core in an unstable manner. If you're tired of doing sit-ups, crunches and reverse sit-ups, and are familiar with other floor-based core exercises, you may welcome the ab wheel.

Many people who use the ab wheel combine it with traditional core exercises to keep their routine fresh and interesting. While all approaches are good, the ab wheel offers a slightly different level of core involvement not seen in other core-exercise devices. In addition, depending on the exercise you do, you could also tone your upper or lower body at the same time.

One of the ab wheel's main goals is to improve core stability, which some researchers claim can improve sports performance in tennis and golf. It's believed that if the core is solid, it can transfer force up and down the kinetic chain, from the upper extremities to the ground or vice versa. A solid core has also been shown to improve posture and reduce lower back strain.

If you're looking to get a defined six-pack stomach, however, know that you'll need to get down to a very lean body weight in addition to working your core. Unfortunately, doing just sit-ups, crunches and even the ab wheel won't get you there. On the other hand, if you use the ab wheel, eat healthily and get plenty of aerobic exercise, you'll be pleased to notice your midsection getting firmer, your posture improving and your appearance looking more slender and fit.

The Core
The torso of the human body is commonly referred to as the "core" because the core of anything is generally the most important element of that thing, whether it's the core of an apple or the core of a nuclear reac-

tor. Although no one universal definition of what constitutes the "core" exists, it's often agreed that the core consists of the abdominal muscles in the front, the muscles of the back that run up and down the spine and sometimes the gluteal region.

The abdominal muscles play a significant role in activities of daily living, including walking and sitting. The ab wheel assists you in building a solid infrastructure to hold you up tall. It does this by engaging the numerous muscles around your midsection, as if you're creating your own corset. Having a strong, stable core is believed to improve posture and enhance the effectiveness of functional and athletic movements. Training the core is more than doing a bunch of sit-ups or crunches; it's an integrated approach of decreasing muscle imbalances that includes flexibility work and mindful conditioning.

I think of the core muscles as guide wires trying to keep a tall pole erect. If one set of wires is too tight and the others too lax, the pole won't be stable. The same thing occurs in people who don't have proper symmetrical alignment. Correct core training is about body awareness and proper activation of specific muscles at specific times to function properly in a coordinated fashion, even when you're not thinking about your core, such as when hitting a baseball or tennis ball, swinging a golf club or lifting something up.

Some experts maintain that true core training is critical for all people. In most physical activities, force needs to be transferred through the body. If the core is "soft" like a limp noodle, energy is lost. That minimal loss can make a difference in the power of your tennis serve or golf swing, or even whether you strain your back muscles or not. This book provides exercises that engage the total kinetic chain of muscles, from the neck to the ankles. Just like every floor in a building is critical to the stability of the building, every segment of the body is critical to the level above and below.

Some of the benefits of having a stable core are:

- Reduced back problems
- Improved athletic performance
- Reduced fatigue
- Improved posture

The Muscles

The muscles on the anterior side of the body provide a great number of critical functions, which include supporting and protecting the internal organs and assisting in proper posture. The muscles of the core are very complex and have different shapes and functions. It's important for us to understand the location and function of these muscles to truly grasp the essence of core training.

The major players included in the core muscle group are transverse abdominis, rectus abdominis, internal and external obliques, and erector spinae group; some circles include the gluteus muscle group. The chart below and the following descriptions will give you a basic under-

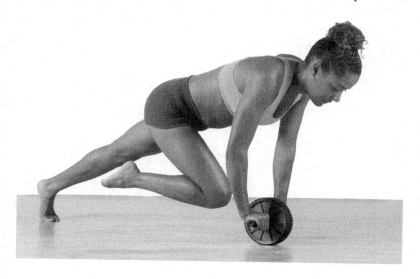

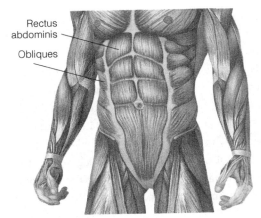

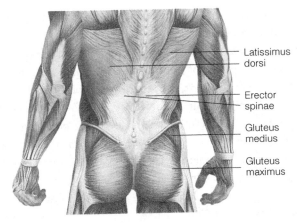

Major Muscles of the Core

standing of the location and role of each muscle.

Transverse Abdominis: The deepest fibers of the abdominal wall, the function of this is to provide support for the internal organs and assist with maintaining proper posture. A good way to engage the transverse abdominis is to "draw the belly button in."

Rectus Abdominis: Best known in fitness circles as the "six pack," this muscle is the most superficial of the core group. It's most generally exercised when doing flexion exercises of the spine, such as sit-ups. Some of its lesser-known duties include stabilizing the pelvis during walking and providing intra-abdominal pressure.

Internal and External Obliques: Found on the sides of the torso, these muscles are engaged to rotate the torso. They can also assist in flexing the vertebral column and providing compression of the abdominal wall. The obliques get activated when you swing a golf club or play tennis.

Erector Spinae Group: The prime movers when extending the back (or bringing you upright from a bent-over position), the erector spinae group also adds trunk stability and helps maintain proper posture. This group of muscles includes the iliocostalis, the longissimus and the spinalis muscles. Each muscle originates and terminates at a different point along the back of the spine, which is why it's called the erector spinae group. Lying on your back and lifting your rear end off the ground is a basic method to engage this muscle group.

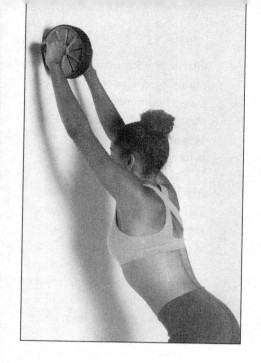

the ab wheel's role in posture

Poor posture and chronic misuse of the back can lead to lower back pain, which affects up to 80 percent of Americans. Back pain is second only to the common cold for time lost from work. For some people poor posture is the result of structural defects, but for most people poor posture is the result of functional abuse over time, such as hunching over a desk all day or incorrectly bending and lifting. Maintaining proper posture can make a significant difference in long-term upper and lower back health.

Proper posture entails the correct balance between opposing muscle groups and correct alignment of the neck and spine. Keeping proper posture is a 24/7 job. We need to be mindful of our posture whether we're standing, sitting or lying down. When we're aligned properly, our joints are in a state of balance wherein the muscles are exerting the least amount of strain to keep us upright.

Our spines, along with the cushioning components known as discs, are pretty hardy. Most people don't hurt their backs with just one bad move—chronic misuse is the culprit. I like to think the spine is like a paper clip. Bend the paper clip once or twice and it still remains strong, but continually bend and twist it and it eventually snaps. The same holds true for our spine. When we chronically engage in poor biomechanical activities, over time the structures around the spine yield to the stresses and break down, which often leads to

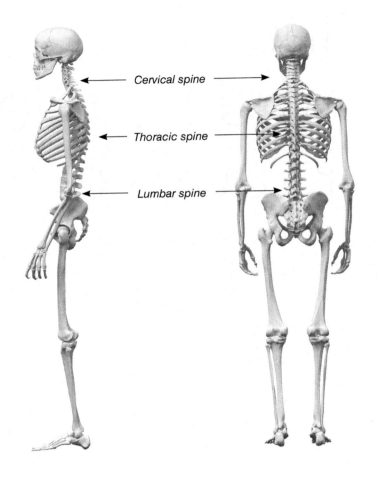

Cervical spine

Thoracic spine

Lumbar spine

lower back injuries. This is why so often we hear people say they were just bending over to pick up a newspaper when their back went out. It's not that one movement that caused the problem but all the previous times that happened before it. Thus it's the proverbial straw that broke the back!

Maintaining good core muscle strength and endurance and engaging in proper body mechanics lowers your risk of having chronic lower back pain. The

Spine Team is made up of a pole called the vertebral column and guide wires called the muscles.

The vertebral spine is designed in a manner to provide optimal function and has three natural curves. The cervical spine (the neck) curves slightly forward. The middle portion of the spine (thoracic spine) curves outward. The lower back (lumbar spine) curves inward. Optimally, the pressures in and around the lower back region and pelvis are evenly

distributed. Sometimes as a result of misuse, disuse or abuse, these curves become misaligned. When the spinal unit is misaligned, we set ourselves up for chronic back pain.

The postural muscles are designed for prolonged work, such as holding the human torso erect. The role of torso muscles is to not fatigue when held in a static position. As stated earlier, the torso muscles need to engage properly so that the arms and legs have a solid platform from which to operate.

As with any guide-wire system, if one set is too tight and the other is slack, alignment issues arise. In most humans there is a significant mal-alignment in their muscles, with some being too tight and others too weak. As Joseph Pilates said years ago, stretch what is tight and strengthen what is slack. Nothing could be truer than that when it comes to core training.

On an aesthetic note, if you want to look more slender or healthier, good posture is the answer. Just stand as you normally do, then stand erect with your shoulders back and chest out. Look at what happens to your belly. Good posture makes us look healthier and skinnier in addition to decreasing lower back discomfort.

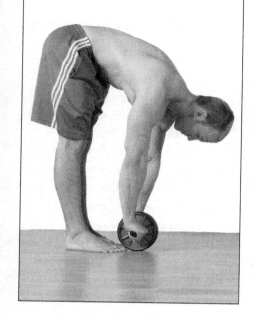

before you begin

Ab wheel training is as easy as just rolling along to a firm and fit abdominal area. However, as with any exercise device, always make sure you're healthy enough to engage in such training by consulting with your health professional first. If you have lower back concerns, hypertension, abdominal strains, or shoulder or wrist joint issues, be prudent in your use of this type of training.

All too often people in their rush to get fit overtrain and injure themselves, especially when it involves a new fitness toy. Train, don't strain! Always underestimate your ability. There is a term in exercise physiology called "specificity of training." While you may be in shape in one skill, that fitness may not transfer over to another. Therefore, even if you have abs of steel and can crank out 100 sit-ups, this may not mean you can't overdo ab wheel training. Train smart, not hard! Introduce one to two exercises at a time, do the minimal amount of reps or duration and move on from there. Amend your routine periodically to avoid getting stale and in order to challenge your body in various ways.

Ab Wheel Training Tips

Using the ab wheel requires total mind-body interaction. Just pounding out sit-ups to the latest tunes is not what core stabilization training is all about. In addition, sloppy and careless movements cause injury. Every movement needs to be performed with a neutral spine. Consider turning off the music and focusing on engaging the proper muscles for the exercise. Teach your mind to engage the core muscles automatically so everything is placed in muscle memory for everyday use.

Because it will take some time for your body to learn how to properly engage your core muscles while moving the wheel, don't expect quick results. With proper mindful training, your core will learn when to contract and when to release in the most efficient manner. Slow and steady wins the core training race. Ripped abdominal muscles don't mean that a person has a strong and solid core. All the muscles of the back, sides and front need to have the correct amount of muscular endurance, strength and flexibility to perform smoothly.

Here are some other things to keep in mind for a safe, effective workout with your ab wheel.

- The ab wheel can and should be used daily. If you're pressed for time, work the front side of your body one day and then the posterior side of your body the next.
- Avoid doing core exercises in the morning because it's believed that intervertebral fluid pressure in the spinal region is higher first thing in the morning.
- Focus on endurance of the core muscles rather than aiming to make the muscles overly strong.
- Don't hold your breath while performing the exercises.
- Practice quality of movement over quantity. More is not better. Only perfect practice makes perfect!
- Slowly progress to more challenging movements.
- All plank exercises are extremely challenging. Make sure you can do the kneeling versions of these exercises before progressing to the plank.

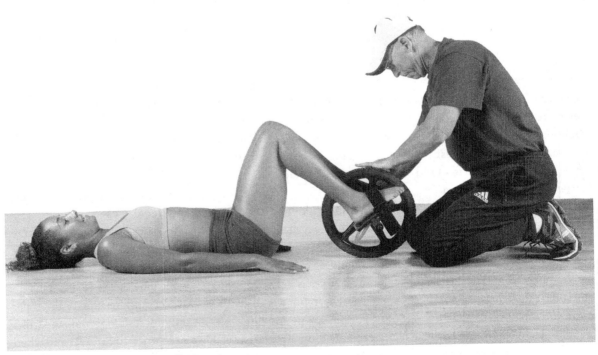

Author Karl Knopf makes some adjustments.

PART 2

programs

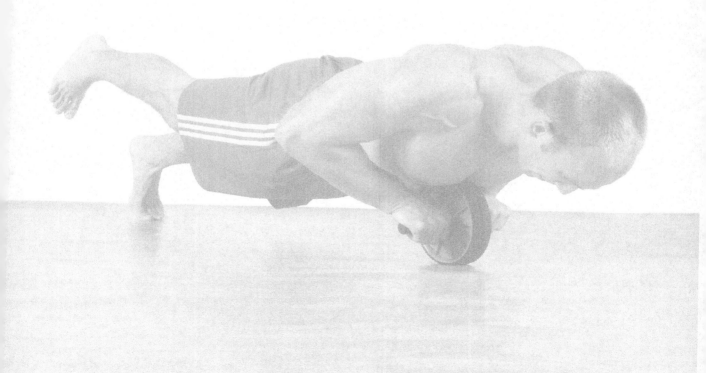

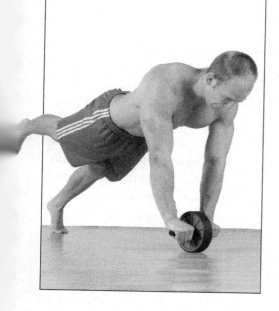

how to use this book

There are several ways you can approach this book: Follow one of the workouts starting on "Beginner Level 1" on page 21, or design your own workout by choosing from the exercises featured in Part 3. Regardless of your fitness level, if you haven't used an ab wheel before, it's prudent to start at the beginner level.

Starting at the basic level allows you to learn and feel how your body reacts to the movements and then place that knowledge in your muscle memory. If you're fit, you'll progress through each level quickly until you reach a level that really challenges you. If you do too much too soon, you'll likely strain muscles, get upset and think that the author is an idiot.

Once you've done a light warm-up (gentle walk, light jog, jumping jacks) to prepare your body for movement, you can start your ab wheel exercises. Stay focused and in the moment. This will help you to keep control during every phase of the movement. For best results (and to keep your back safe), you should also move your torso (shoulders, hips, spine) as one unit. Always realign your spine, if necessary, after each rep. Try not to "cheat" by using muscles other than the ones you should be targeting. In fact, the more athletic you are, the more easily you'll be able to recruit muscles other than those intended to do the work. Cheating reduces the effective of the exercise and can be potentially unsafe for your body.

Remember that you're not competing with anyone. You don't need to complete all the exercises in any given workout in a certain amount of time. When your body has had enough, listen to it. However, if you feel like you could do more, you can add the bonus exercise(s) at the end of each workout. After your workout, finish up with some stretching (see page 77 for ideas) to reduce any soreness you might have later.

Designing Your Own Workout
The exercises in Part 3 are grouped according to the position in which they're done: supine (on your back), hands and knees, plank, prone (on your front) and against the wall. This should make it easy for you to select your

exercises should you decide to design your own workouts.

Keep in mind that there's no ideal set of exercises. Your ab wheel routine needs to evolve and adapt to your goals and fitness level. Some people will be doing ab wheel exercises for rehabilitative purposes, some for general fitness, and others to enhance appearance. Therefore, use your inner wisdom when selecting exercises for your ab wheel workout. Perhaps you'll have a set of exercises to do on Mondays, a different set on Wednesdays, and yet another set on Fridays.

You can also let your mood determine your selection for the day. If you're rushed for time,

one day perform movements that focus on the backside of your core, while another day work the front side. Don't get so locked into a routine that you lose spontaneity and look for excuses to avoid the work. Aim for 5–15 minutes of ab wheel training daily, or at least every other day. Be creative yet safe and avoid overtraining.

When you're first beginning, a rest period of 30 seconds to 1 minute between sets should be adequate. However, the key is not to overstrain the abdominal region. A strained abdominal muscle is very uncomfortable and can take a while to heal, thus be cautious and focused, resting as needed. As you become more fit,

you may shorten the rest time between sets. If you find yourself getting sore or overfatigued, perform moves every other day.

Your body will tell you when to add a new move or step up to the next level. Unlike weight training, ab wheel training is subtle, working the deep-lying muscles of the body that support and stabilize the core. Kneeling or supine exercises are generally a safe way to start. However, each of us is unique so if something doesn't feel right, experiment until you find moves that resonate with your body. If your body feels best while doing supine exercises, then go for it!

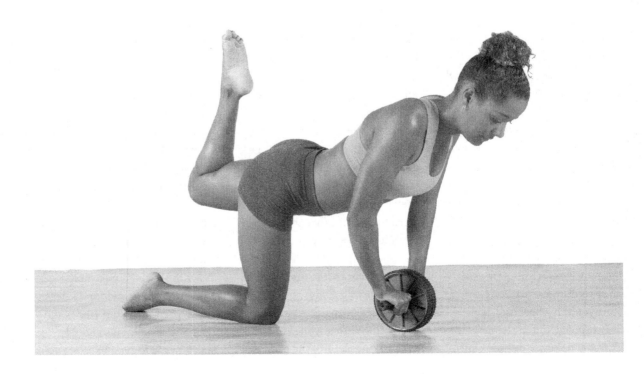

Beginner Level 1

This routine is for folks who are new to core exercise and just starting a fitness program. Perform 1 set of 5 reps or hold static moves 5–10 seconds. Never hold your breath.

BEGINNER LEVEL 1

Warm up for at least 10 minutes and stretch after your workout. See pages 77–86 for suggestions.

EXERCISE	SETS	REP/TIME	REST
Basic Foundational Position *page 29*	1	5	:30–:60
Mad Cat *page 41*	1	5	:30–:60
Kneeling Push-Up *page 49*	1	5	:30–:60
Wall Plank *page 74*	1	:05–:10	:30–:60
Shoulder Roll-Down *page 73*	1	5	:30–:60
Supine Arm Swing *page 30*	1	5	:30–:60
Supine Fly *page 31*	1	5	:30–:60
I's, Y's & T's *page 32*	1	5	:30–:60
Heel Slide *page 33*	1	5	:30–:60
Curl-Up *page 34*	1	5	:30–:60
Pelvic Lift *page 38*	1	5	:30–:60
Bonus: Roll-Out *page 46*	1	5	:30–:60

Beginner Level 2

Do not progress to this level unless you can easily perform all the Beginner Level 1 movements with perfect form. Perform 1 set of 10 reps or hold static moves 5–15 seconds. Never hold your breath.

BEGINNER LEVEL 2

Warm up for at least 10 minutes and stretch after your workout. See pages 77–86 for suggestions.

EXERCISE	SETS	REP/TIME	REST
Forward Shoulder Roll-Up *page 70*	1	10	:30–:60
Reverse Shoulder Roll-Up *page 71*	1	10	:30–:60
Wall Push-Up *page 75*	1	10	:30–:60
Stork Stand Roll-Up *page 76*	1	10	:30–:60
Pelvic Lift with Arm Lift *page 39*	1	10	:30–:60
Alternating Curl-Up *page 35*	1	10	:30–:60
Supine Arm Swing *page 30*	1	10	:30–:60
Feet to Hands *page 59*	1	10	:30–:60
Kneeling Push-Up *page 49*	1	10	:30–:60
Child's Pose *page 42*	1	:05–:15	:30–:60
Bonus: Hands to Feet *page 58*	1	10	:30–:60

Intermediate Level 1

Once you can achieve perfect form in the previous series you're ready to progress to this level. If you push yourself too fast and too soon, you're setting yourself up for injury and failure. The best results are achieved when done correctly.

Perform 1 set of 5–10 reps or hold static moves 5–10 seconds. Never hold your breath.

INTERMEDIATE LEVEL 1

Warm up for at least 10 minutes and stretch after your workout. See pages 77–86 for suggestions.

EXERCISE	SETS	REP/TIME	REST
Wall Plank *page 74*	1	:05–:10	:30
Wall V Roll-Up *page 72*	1	5–10	:30
Single-Leg Lift *page 65*	1	5–10/side	:30
Shoulder Extender *page 63*	1	5–10	:30
Reverse Shoulder Extender *page 40*	1	5–10	:30
Pelvic Lift with Arm Lift *page 39*	1	5–10	:30
Alternating Curl-Up *page 35*	1	5–10	:30
One-Legged Push-Up *page 61*	1	5–10	:30
Plank to Pike *page 60*	1	5–10	:30
Donkey Kick *page 50*	1	5–10	:30
Bonus: Plank *page 53*	1	:05–:10	:30

Intermediate Level 2

This is only to be done once you can easily perform all the Intermediate Level 1 movements with perfect form. Perform 2 set of 15 reps or hold static moves 10–20 seconds. Never hold your breath.

INTERMEDIATE LEVEL 2

Warm up for at least 10 minutes and stretch after your workout. See pages 77–86 for suggestions.

EXERCISE	SETS	REP/TIME	REST
Child's Pose *page 42*	2	:10–:20	:30
Pointer Sequence *page 43*	2	15	:30
Half Roll-Out *page 45*	2	15	:30
Kickback *page 55*	2	15	:30
Fire Hydrant *page 51*	2	15	:30
One-Legged Plank *page 56*	2	:10–:20/side	:30
V Roll-Out *page 47*	2	15	:30
Supine Fly *page 31*	2	15	:30
Curl-Up *page 34*	2	15	:30
Pelvic Lift with Arm Lift *page 39*	2	15	:30
Bonus: Roll-Out *page 46*	2	15	:30

Advanced

This workout is designed for those with an above-average level of fitness and good body control. Perform 3 sets of 15 reps. Never hold your breath.

ADVANCED

Warm up for at least 10 minutes and stretch after your workout. See pages 77–86 for suggestions.

EXERCISE	SETS	REP/TIME	REST
Wrist Stretch *page 44*	3	15	:30
One-Legged Roll-Out *page 48*	3	15/side	:30
Push-Up *page 57*	3	15	:30
Leg Curl *page 52*	3	15	:30
Plank to Pike *page 60*	3	15	:30
Heel Slide *page 33*	3	15	:30
Hold/Relax Curl-Up *page 36*	3	15	:30
Supine Leg Press-Out *page 37*	3	15	:30
Shoulder Extender *page 63*	3	15	:30
Double-Leg Lift *page 67*	3	15	:30
Bonus: One-Legged Plank *page 56*	3	:10–:20/side	:30
Bonus: Combo Arm & Leg Lift *page 66*	3	15	:30

Super-Fit

This set of exercises is designed for folks who are extremely fit and have excellent body control and awareness. Do not do this set of exercises unless you're in excellent shape and great health. Make sure you warm up well before performing these moves; stretch afterward. Perform 2–3 sets of 15–20 reps. Never hold your breath.

SUPER-FIT

Warm up for at least 10 minutes and stretch after your workout. See pages 77–86 for suggestions.

EXERCISE	SETS	REP/TIME	REST
Pointer Sequence *page 43*	2–3	15–20	:15–:30
V Roll-Out *page 47*	2–3	15–20	:15–:30
One-Legged Roll-Out *page 48*	2–3	15–20/side	:15–:30
Leg Curl *page 52*	2–3	15–20	:15–:30
Leg Abduction & Adduction *page 54*	2–3	15–20	:15–:30
One-Legged Plank *page 56*	2–3	alap*/side	:15–:30
Plank to Pike *page 60*	2–3	15–20	:15–:30
One-Legged Push-Up *page 61*	2–3	15–20	:15–:30
Curl-Up *page 34*	2–3	15–20	:15–:30
Superhero *page 64*	2–3	15–20	:15–:30
Bonus: Double-Double *page 68*	2–3	15–20	:15–:30
Bonus: Plank Roll-Out *page 62*	2–3	15–20	:15–:30
Super-Fit Bonus: Pop-Up *page 69*	2–3	15–20	:15–:30

* as long as possible

PART 3

the

exercises

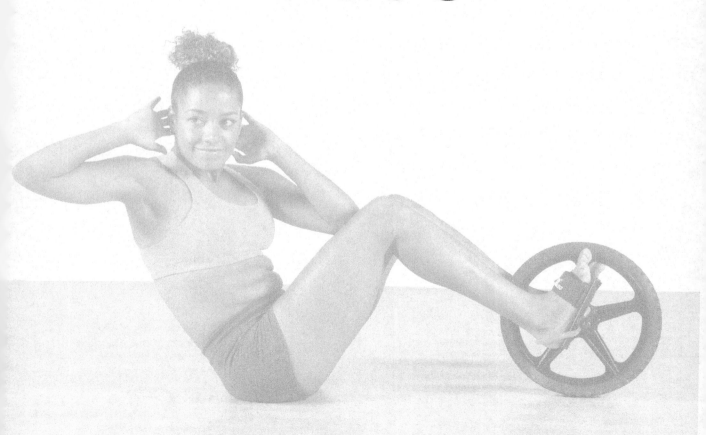

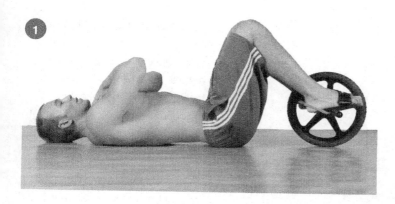

This exercise helps you gain awareness of core muscles and learn proper posture while performing supine wheel exercises.

1 Lie on your back with your knees bent and feet inserted in the wheel straps.

2 Contract your abdominals and slowly push the small of your back into the floor—pretend that you're trying to compress a sponge that's under the small of your back. Hold for 10 seconds.

Release and allow the small of your back to return to neutral.

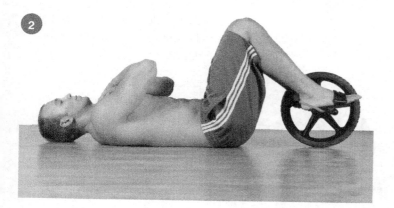

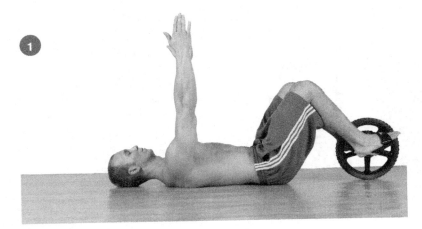

1 Lie on your back with your knees bent and feet inserted in the wheel straps. Extend both arms to the ceiling, with palms facing each other. Make sure to maintain neutral spine throughout the movement.

2 Slowly move one arm forward toward the hip and the other straight back toward your ear. Hold for a moment.

Slowly return to starting position, then move your arms the other direction.

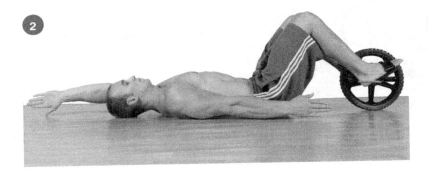

VARIATION: Hold weights for an extra challenge.

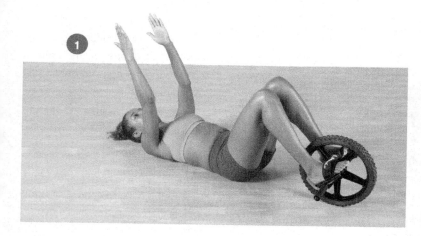

1 Lie on your back with your knees bent and feet inserted in the wheel straps. Extend both arms to the ceiling, with palms facing each other. Make sure to maintain neutral spine throughout the movement.

2 Slowly open your arms to the sides. Hold and relax.

Slowly return to starting position.

VARIATION: Hold weights for an extra challenge.

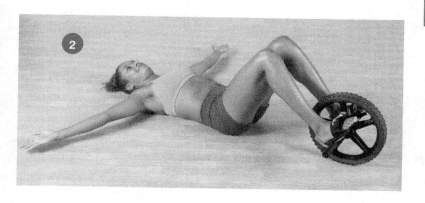

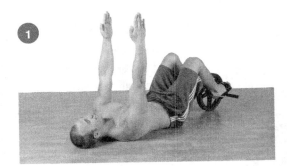

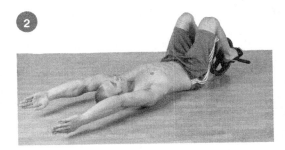

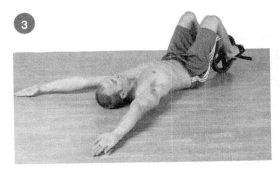

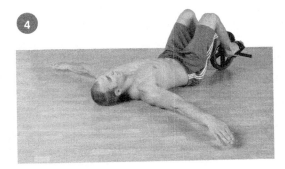

1 Lie on your back with your knees bent and feet inserted in the wheel straps. Extend both arms to the ceiling, with palms facing each other. Make sure to maintain neutral spine throughout the movement.

2 Slowly and deliberately take both arms over your head and toward the floor, making your body look like an "I" from a bird's eye view.

3 Return to starting position and then slightly open your arms to the sides and to the floor as if making a "Y."

4 Return to starting position and then open your arms wide and lower your knuckles to the floor to make a "T."

VARIATION: Hold weights for an extra challenge.

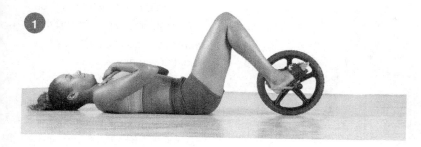

This exercise is easier to perform when done on a smooth floor surface. The focus of this exercise is to not allow the lower back to arch. Only move your heels out as far as you can while still keeping your back neutral.

1 Lie on your back with your knees bent and feet inserted in the wheel straps. Make sure to maintain neutral spine throughout the movement.

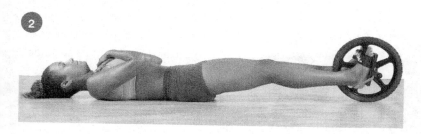

2 While keeping your core engaged, slowly and mindfully slide your feet forward along the floor.

Return to starting position.

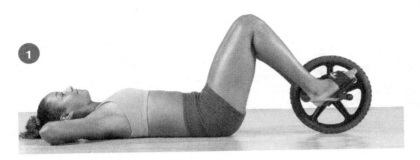

Focus on pressing your lower back into the floor and performing this correctly, not quickly. Don't worry about how many you can do.

1 Lie on your back with your knees bent and feet inserted in the wheel straps. Place your hands behind your head to cradle and support your neck.

2 Inhale, tuck your chin to your chest and exhale while slowly lifting your shoulder blades off the floor, contracting your abdominal muscles. Hold for 1 to 3 seconds.

Inhale and slowly return to starting position.

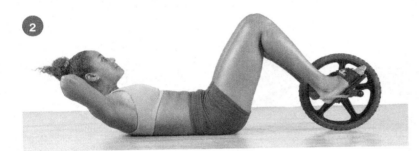

ADVANCED VARIATION: You can also curl up all the way.

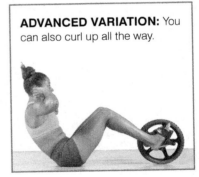

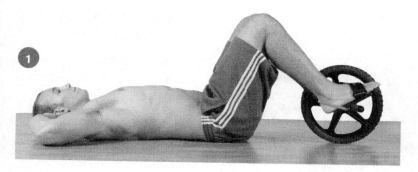

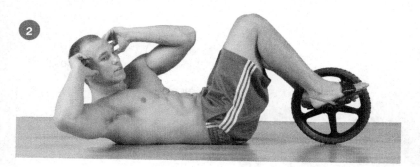

Focus on pressing your lower back into the floor and performing this correctly, not quickly. Don't worry about how many you can do.

1 Lie on your back with your knees bent and feet inserted in the wheel straps. Place your hands behind your head to cradle and support your neck.

2 Inhale, tuck your chin to your chest, exhale while slowly lifting your shoulder blades off the floor, and twist your torso to bring your left elbow toward your right knee. Hold for 1 to 3 seconds.

Inhale and slowly return to starting position. Repeat to the opposite side. Continue alternating.

ADVANCED VARIATION: You can also curl up all the way or bring your lower legs up 90 degrees and perform the movement.

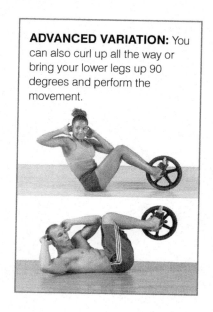

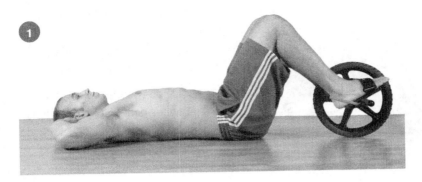

Focus on pressing your lower back into the floor.

1 Lie on your back with your knees bent and feet inserted in the wheel straps.

2 Inhale, tuck your chin to your chest, slowly lifting your shoulder blades off the floor. Now twist your torso gently and then exhale while pressing your left hand into your right knee. Hold for 1 to 3 seconds.

Slowly return to starting position.

Repeat, then switch sides.

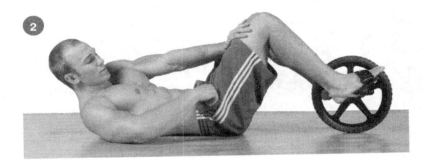

VARIATION: This can also be done with your knees bent 90 degrees.

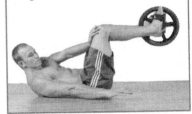

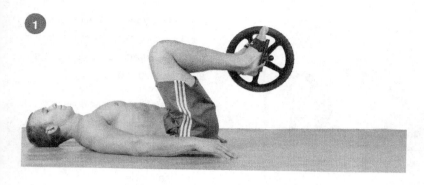

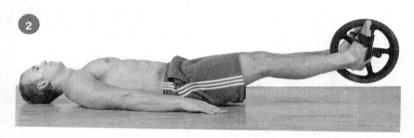

Caution: Do not do this if you have a history of sway back or lower back pain.

1 Lie on your back with your feet inserted in the wheel straps and knees bent 90 degrees. Rest your arms alongside your body.

2 Maintaining proper core stability, slowly extend your legs forward, keeping them a few inches off the floor.

Return to starting position.

SUPINE SERIES
pelvic lift

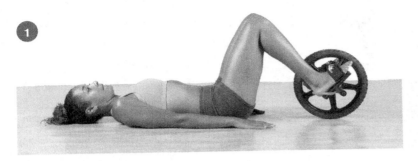

1 Lie on your back with your knees bent and feet inserted in the wheel straps. Rest your arms alongside your body.

2 Press both feet equally into the floor, causing your pelvis to lift off the floor. Do not lift your butt so high as to arch your back. Hold for 3 to 5 seconds.

Slowly lower to the floor. Realign your spine after each rep.

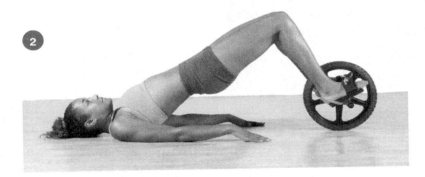

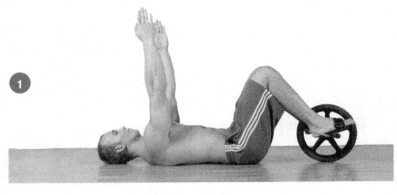

1 Lie on your back with your knees bent and feet inserted in the wheel straps. Extend both arms up to the ceiling, with your palms facing each other.

2 Press both feet equally into the floor, causing your pelvis to lift off the floor. Do not lift your butt so high that it causes you to arch your back. Hold for 3 to 5 seconds.

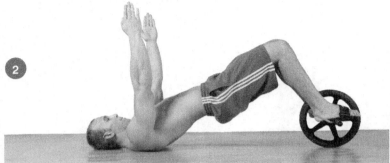

3 Slowly move one arm forward toward your hip and the other straight back by your ear.

4 Slowly extend yours arms back up to the ceiling and then switch directions.

Repeat then slowly lower to the floor.

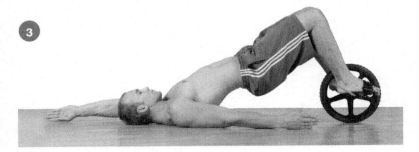

VARIATION: Hold weights for an extra challenge.

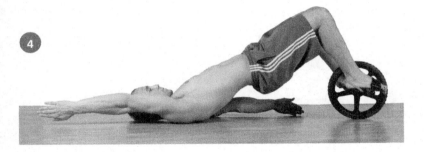

SUPINE SERIES
reverse shoulder extender

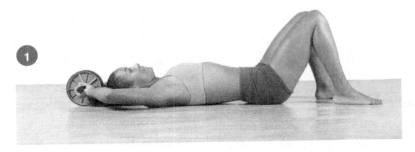

1 Lie on your back with your knees bent. Grasp the handles of the wheel with both hands and place the wheel on the ground just above your head.

2 Slowly extend your arms along the floor.

Return to starting position, realigning your spine after each rep.

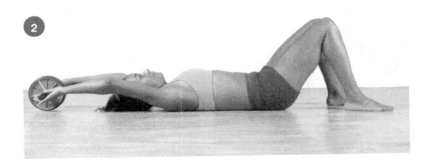

This exercise aims to improve lower back flexibility.

1 Get on your hands and knees with your hands on the wheel.

2 Inhale and pull your belly button in, causing your back to round.

As you exhale, slowly relax your body to return to starting position.

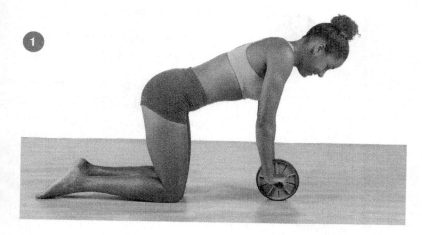

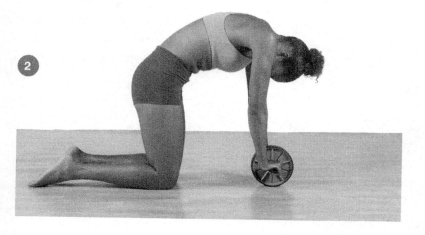

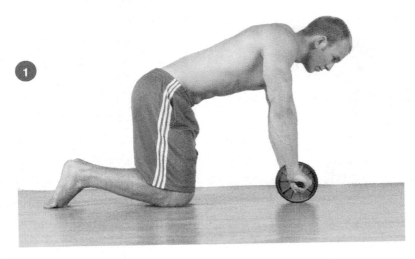

This exercise aims to improve lower back flexibility.

1 Get on your hands and knees with your hands on the wheel.

2 Rest your butt on your heels and roll the wheel forward as far as you can while still maintaining proper neutral spine.

Roll the wheel back to starting position. Hold and relax your back.

> **MODIFICATION:** This can also be performed with your knees resting on a rolled-up towel.

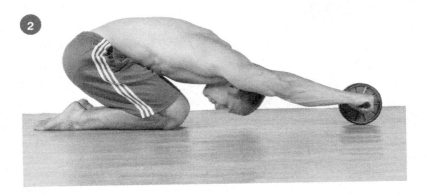

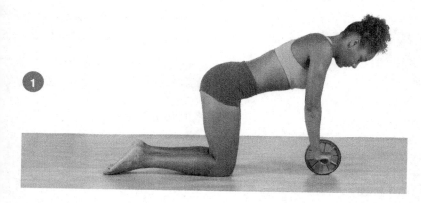

This is a good balance and core stability builder.

1 Get on your hands and knees with your hands on the wheel.

2 Once you're stable and stationary, raise and extend your right leg behind you. Hold.

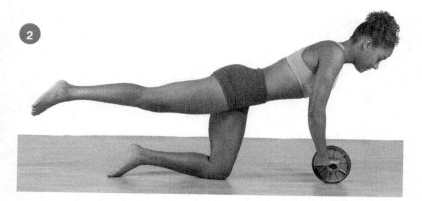

3 Lower it slowly and raise and extend your left leg. Hold.

Lower it slowly and continue alternating legs.

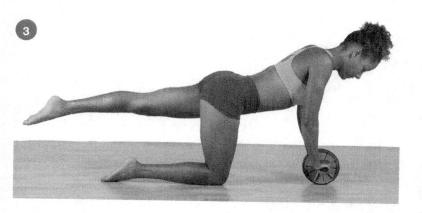

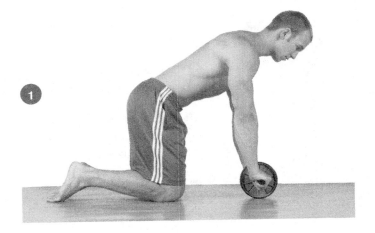

1 Get on your hands and knees with your hands on the wheel.

2 Slowly roll your knuckles forward and downward. Hold.

3 Roll your knuckles backward.

Slowly continue to roll your knuckles downward and backward.

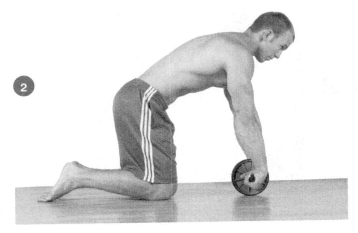

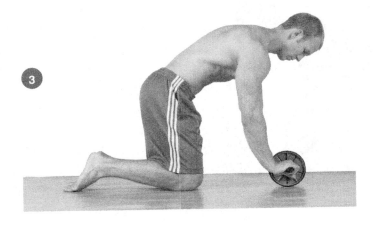

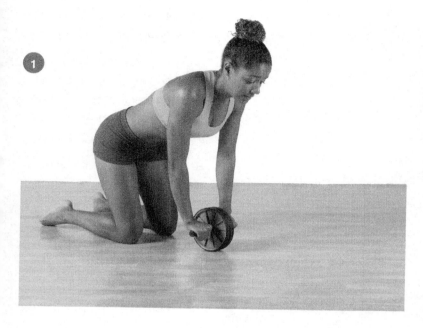

1 Get on your hands and knees with your hands on the wheel.

2 Slowly roll the wheel forward about 12 inches or so, maintaining proper form. Hold for a moment.

Return to starting position and realign your posture.

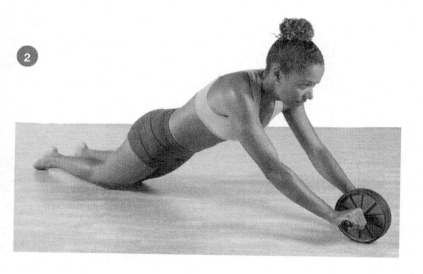

KNEELING SERIES
roll-out

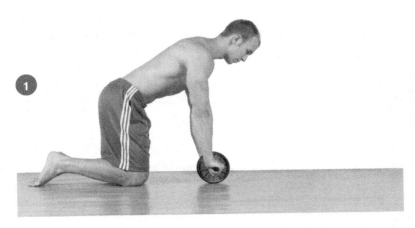

1 Get on your hands and knees with your hands on the wheel.

2 Slowly roll the wheel forward, only going as far as you can control proper form (do not allow your back to sag). Hold for a moment.

Return to starting position and realign your posture.

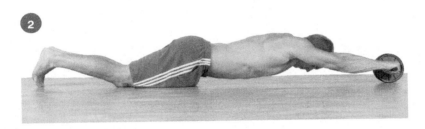

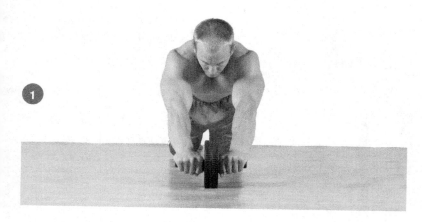

1 Get on your hands and knees with your hands on the wheel.

2 Slowly roll the wheel forward and out to the left, only going as far as you can control proper form (do not allow your back to sag). Hold for a moment.

3 Return to starting position and realign your posture before slowly rolling the wheel forward and out to the right.

Return to starting position.

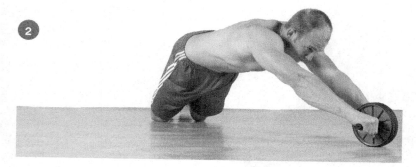

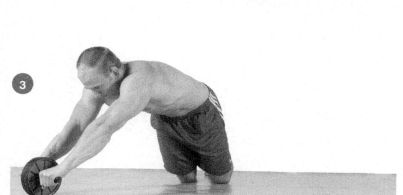

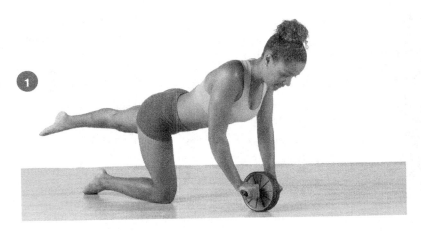

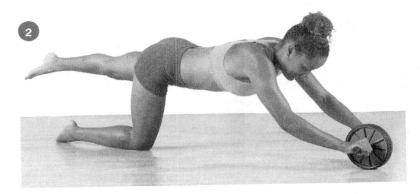

1 Get on your hands and knees with your hands on the wheel. Slowly raise and extend your left leg behind you, balancing on your right knee.

2 Slowly roll the wheel forward, only going as far as you can control proper form (do not allow your back to sag). Hold for a moment.

Roll back to starting position. Finish your reps before switching legs.

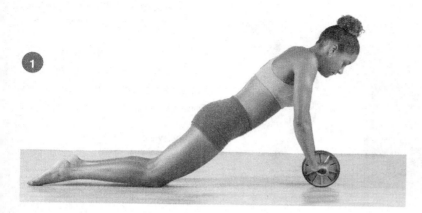

1 Get on your hands and knees with your hands on the wheel. Once you're stable and stationary, roll the wheel forward until you have a nice line from head to knees. Your hands should be in line with your shoulders.

2 Lower your chest to the top of the wheel. Hold for a moment.

Return to starting position and realign your posture.

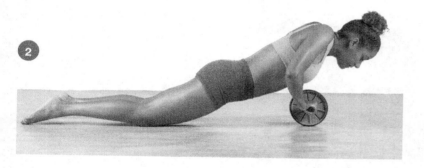

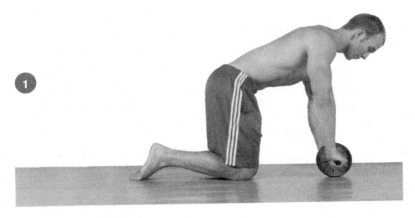

1 Get on your hands and knees with your hands on the wheel.

2 Once you're stable and stationary, draw your right knee toward your right elbow. Hold for a moment.

3 Now extend your leg backward. Hold.

Return to starting position and perform with the other leg. Continue alternating.

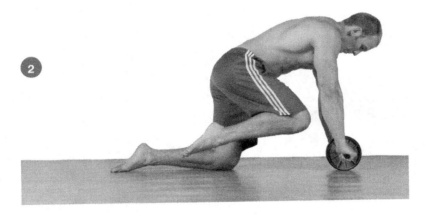

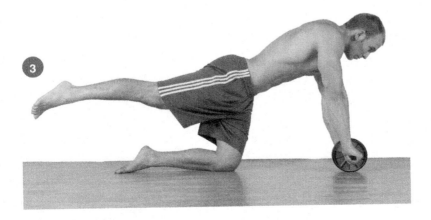

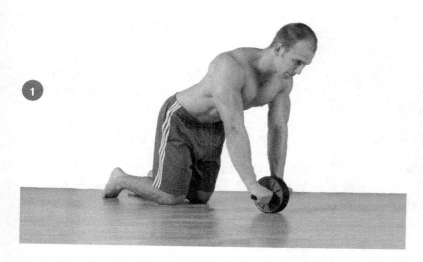

1 Get on your hands and knees with your hands on the wheel.

2 Lift your right leg to the side approximately 90 degrees, if possible.

Return to starting position and perform with your other leg.

> **VARIATION:** Add ankle weights for an extra challenge.

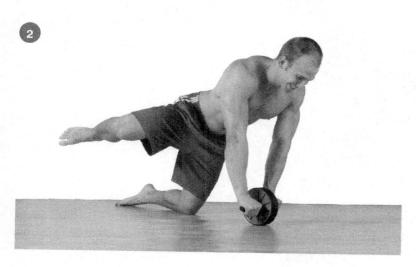

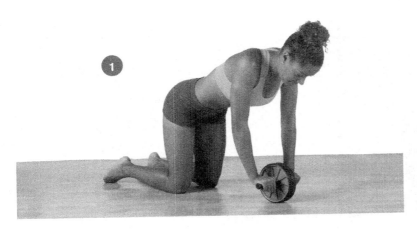

1 Get on your hands and knees with your hands on the wheel.

2 Once you're stable and stationary, lift and straighten your left leg behind you. Hold for a moment.

3 Curl your left leg halfway to your butt.

Straighten the leg and repeat before performing with the other leg.

VARIATION: Add ankle weights for an extra challenge.

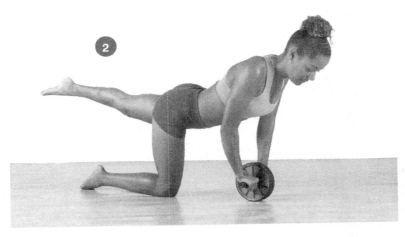

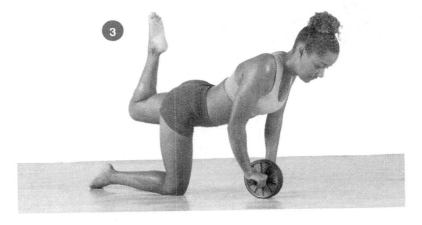

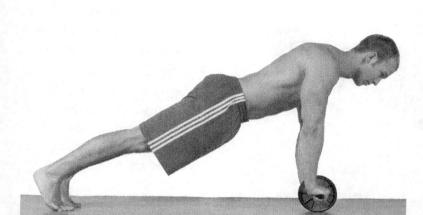

THE POSITION: Get on your hands and knees with your hands on the wheel. Lift your knees off the ground; you may need to walk your feet back until you form a straight line from head to heels. Your hands should be directly under your shoulders. Return your knees to the ground to release.

If you don't have a slider, you may need to wear socks and place your feet on a surface that will allow them to slide.

1 Assume plank position with your hands on the wheel; you should have a straight line from head to heels and your hands should be directly under your shoulders.

2 Slowly slide your left foot out to the side, only going as far as you can maintain perfect posture.

3 Return to starting position then perform with your other leg.

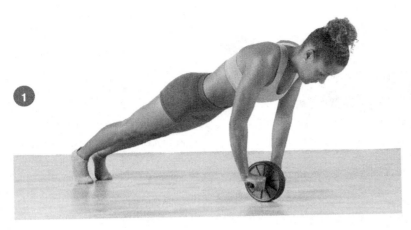

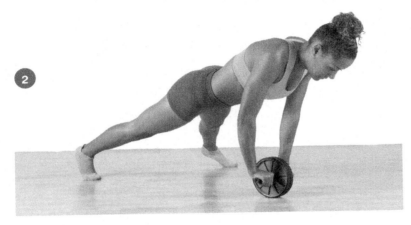

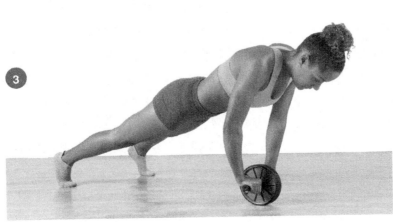

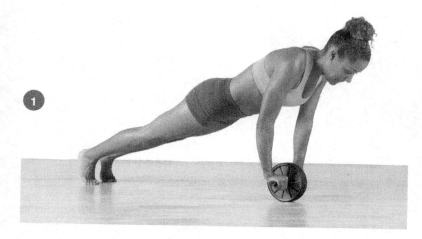

1 Assume plank position with your hands on the wheel; you should have a straight line from head to heels and your hands should be directly under your shoulders.

2 Draw your right knee toward your right elbow. Hold for a moment.

3 Now extend your leg backward. Hold.

Return to starting position and perform with the other leg.

Continue alternating.

> **VARIATION:** Add ankle weights for an extra challenge.

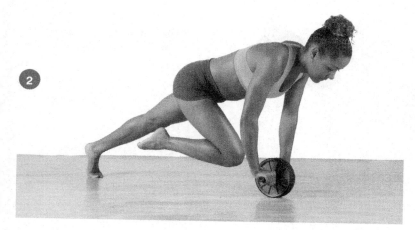

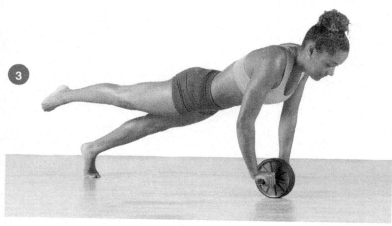

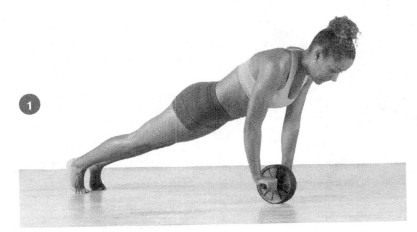

1 Assume plank position with your hands on the wheel; you should have a straight line from head to heels and your hands should be directly under your shoulders.

2 Slowly raise one leg off the ground and hold.

Return your foot to the ground then switch legs to balance out the work.

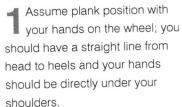

VARIATION: Add ankle weights for an extra challenge.

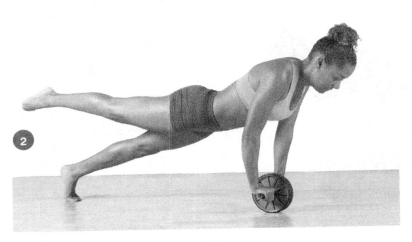

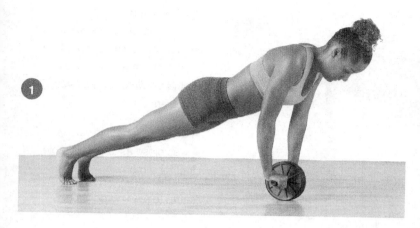

1 Assume plank position with your hands on the wheel; you should have a straight line from head to heels and your hands should be directly under your shoulders.

2 Once you're stable and stationary, lower your chest to the top of the wheel. Hold for a moment.

Return to starting position and realign your posture.

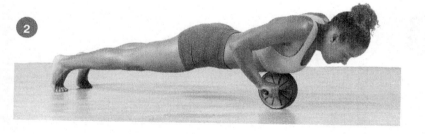

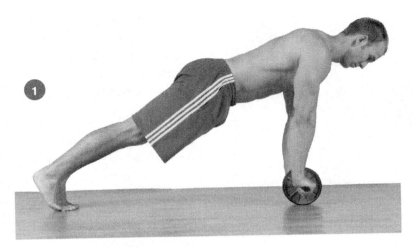

1 Assume plank position with your hands on the wheel; you should have a straight line from head to heels and your hands should be directly under your shoulders.

2 Roll the wheel toward your feet as close as is comfortable. Hold for a moment.

Return to starting position.

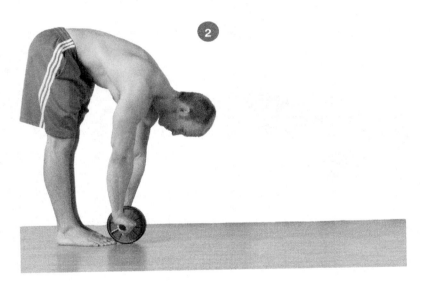

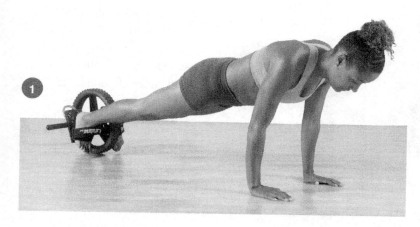

1 Assume plank position with your feet strapped to the wheel; you should have a straight line from head to heels.

2 Keeping your hands in place, roll the wheel toward your hands as close as is comfortable. Hold for a moment.

Return to starting position.

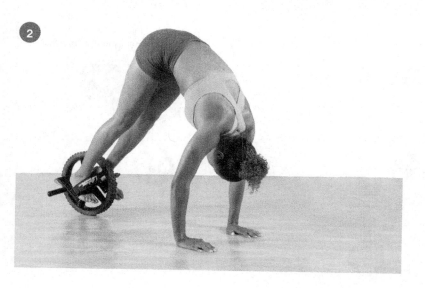

plank to pike

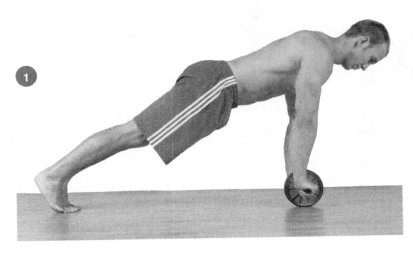

1 Assume plank position with your hands on the wheel; you should have a straight line from head to heels and your hands should be directly under your shoulders.

2 Roll the wheel toward your feet until your body is in a pike (or inverted "V") position.

Return to starting position.

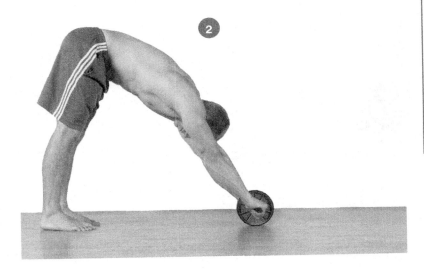

VARIATION: You can also do this exercise with your feet strapped into the ab wheel. Add ankle weights for an extra challenge.

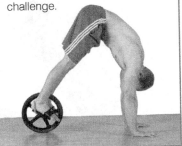

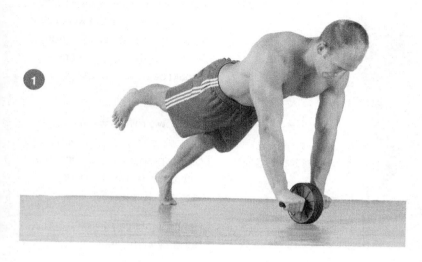

1 Assume plank position with your hands on the wheel; you should have a straight line from head to heels and your hands should be directly under your shoulders. Lift your right leg and hold.

2 Lower your chest to the top of the wheel. Hold for a moment.

Return to starting position, realign your posture and repeat with your other leg up.

Alternate leg lifts as you perform push-ups.

> **VARIATION:** Add ankle weights for an extra challenge.

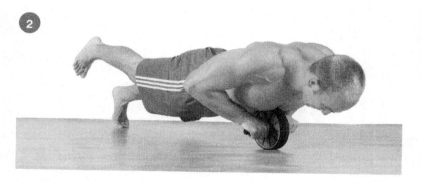

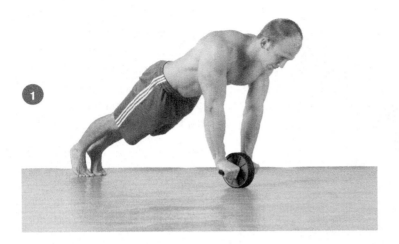

1 Assume plank position with your hands on the wheel; you should have a straight line from head to heels and your hands should be directly under your shoulders.

2 Slowly roll the wheel forward, only going as far as you can control proper form (do not allow your back to sag). Hold for a moment.

Return to starting position and realign your posture.

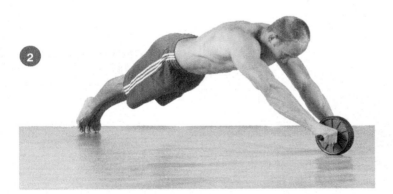

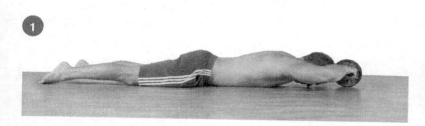

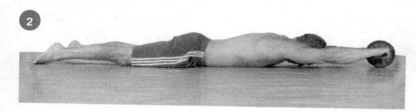

If lying flat is uncomfortable, place a rolled-up towel under your hips.

Caution: If you experience any lower back discomfort, don't lift your extremities much above head height. Stop doing the exercise if pain persists.

1 Lie on your front with your legs extended along the floor. Grasp the handles of the wheel with both hands and place the wheel on the ground just above your head.

2 Slowly extend your arms along the floor.

Return to starting position, realigning your spine after each rep.

PRONE SERIES
superhero

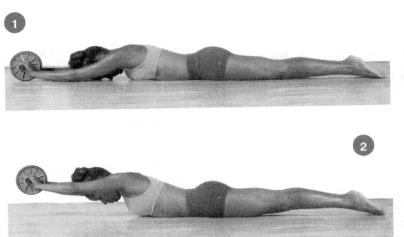

You may find this more comfortable with a rolled-up towel or pillow under your hipbones.

Caution: If you experience any lower back discomfort, don't lift your extremities much above head height. Stop doing the exercise if pain persists.

1 Lie on your front with your arms outstretched forward grasping the wheel handles.

2 Concentrate on maintaining correct alignment and slowly raise both arms. Keep the motion smooth and avoid twisting your body. Hold.

Lower your arms.

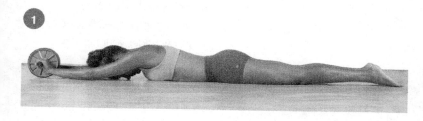

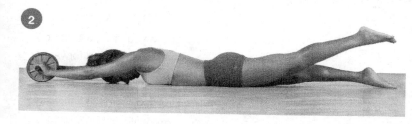

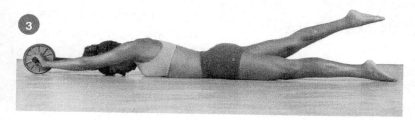

You may find this more comfortable with a rolled-up towel or pillow under your hipbones.

Caution: If you experience any lower back discomfort, don't lift your extremities much above head height. Stop doing the exercise if pain persists.

1 Lie on your front with your arms outstretched forward grasping the wheel handles.

2 Concentrate on maintaining correct alignment and slowly raise one leg. Keep the motion smooth and avoid twisting your body. Hold.

3 Lower and raise the other leg. Hold.

Continue alternating.

VARIATION: To increase leg and butt toning, place ankle weights around your ankles.

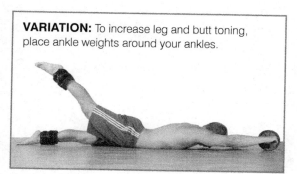

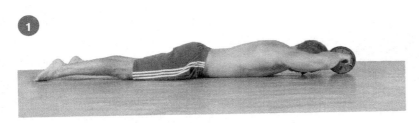

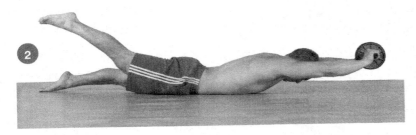

You may find this more comfortable with a rolled-up towel or pillow under your hipbones.

Caution: If you experience any lower back discomfort, don't lift your extremities much above head height. Stop doing the exercise if pain persists.

1 Lie on your front with your arms outstretched forward grasping the wheel handles.

2 Concentrate on maintaining correct alignment while slowly raising both arms and your right leg. Keep the motion smooth and avoid twisting your body. Hold.

Lower your arms and leg, then raise both arms again and your other leg.

VARIATION: To increase leg and butt toning, place ankle weights around your ankles.

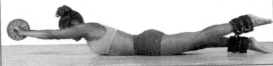

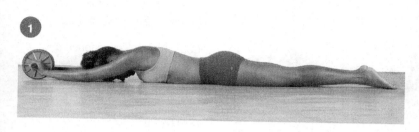

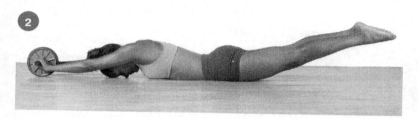

You may find this more comfortable with a rolled-up towel or pillow under your hipbones.

Caution: If you experience any lower back discomfort, don't lift your extremities much above head height. Stop doing the exercise if pain persists.

1 Lie on your front with your arms outstretched forward grasping the wheel handles.

2 Concentrate on maintaining correct alignment while slowly raising both legs. Keep the motion smooth and avoid twisting your body. Hold.

Lower both legs.

VARIATION: To increase leg and butt toning, place ankle weights around your ankles.

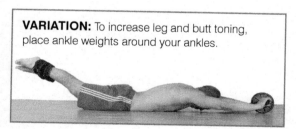

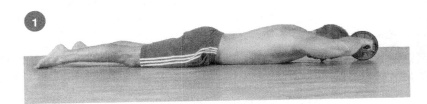

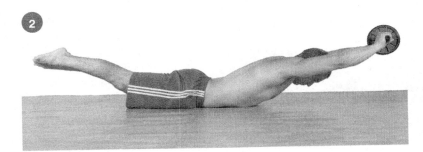

You may find this more comfortable with a rolled-up towel or pillow under your hipbones.

Caution: If you experience any lower back discomfort, don't lift your extremities much above head height. Stop doing the exercise if pain persists.

1 Lie on your front with your arms outstretched forward grasping the wheel handles.

2 Concentrate on maintaining correct alignment while slowly raising both legs and arms. Keep the motion smooth and avoid twisting your body. Hold.

Lower both arms and legs.

VARIATION: To increase leg and butt toning, place ankle weights around your ankles.

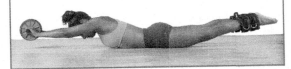

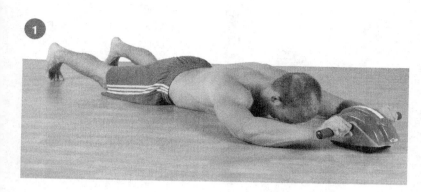

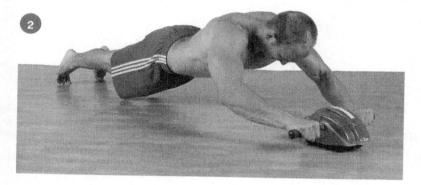

This is an extremely challenging exercise for the fitness elite.

1 Lie on your front and place your hands on the wheel handles and toes on the floor. Stretch your arms and the wheel forward.

2 Roll the wheel approximately 45 to 60 degrees. Now simultaneously apply downward pressure to the wheel and contract your total body to lift your body 1 to 2 inches off the floor.

Release everything to the floor.

forward shoulder roll-up

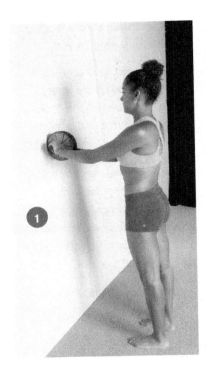

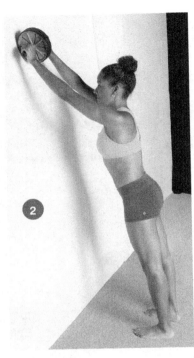

1 Grasping the wheel handles, stand arm's distance from a wall and place the wheel on it at chest height.

2 Slowly roll the wheel as high as is comfortable. Hold.

Roll down to starting position.

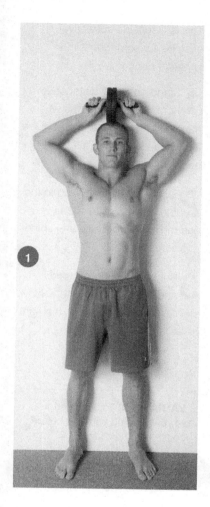

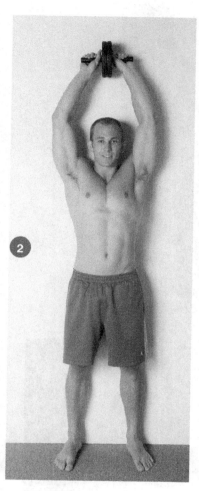

This exercise improves posture by increasing chest and shoulder flexibility.

1 Stand with your back to the wall and attempt to place your head on the wall. Grasping the wheel handles, position the wheel just above your head and hold for 5 to 10 seconds.

2 Roll the wheel as high as you can while keeping your back to the wall.

Return to starting position and realign your posture.

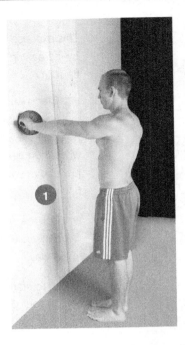

This is a suitable corrective exercise for someone with shoulder concerns.

1 Stand an arm's distance away from the wall, grab the wheel handles with each hand and place the wheel on the wall at chest height.

2 Slowly roll the wheel up to the left, only going as far as you can maintain proper neutral spine position. Hold.

3 Return to starting position and realign your posture. Now slowly roll the wheel up to the right. Hold.

Continue alternating sides.

VARIATION: You can perform all your reps on one side before doing the other side.

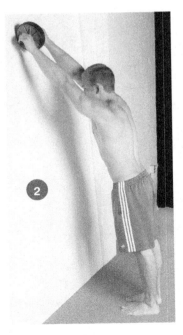

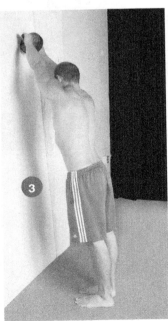

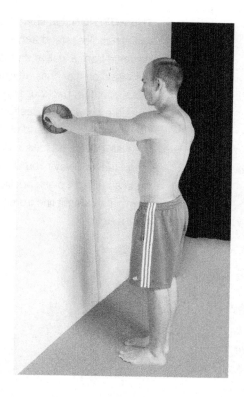

1

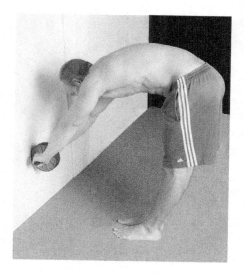

2

Caution: Avoid this exercise if you have a history of lower back problems or high pressure in your eyes.

1 Grasping the wheel handles, stand arm's distance from a wall and place the wheel on it at chest height.

2 Slowly roll the wheel down the wall as close to the floor as is comfortable; keep the pressure against the wall so that the load isn't placed on your lower back. You should feel a gentle stretch in the hamstring muscles in the back of your legs. Hold.

Roll up to starting position.

VARIATION: This can also be done from your knees.

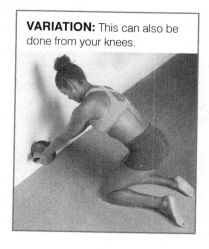

target: upper body, core

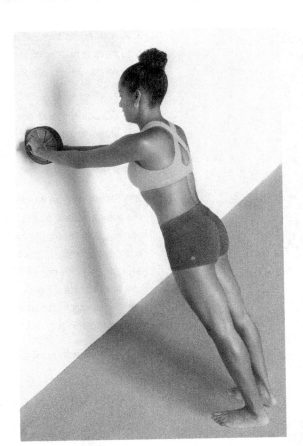

THE POSITION: Grasping the wheel handles, stand arm's distance from a wall and place the wheel on it at chest height. Move your feet backward until your arms are bearing the desired load. (Beginners should stand closer to the wall; advanced folks should stand farther away.) You should be in an upright plank position, forming a straight line from head to heels. Hold.

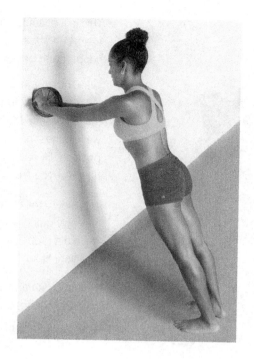

1 Grasping the wheel handles, stand arm's distance from a wall and place the wheel on it at chest height. Move your feet backward until your arms are bearing the desired load. (Beginners should stand closer to the wall; advanced folks should stand farther away.) You should be in an upright plank position, forming a straight line from head to heels.

2 Lower your chest to the wheel.

Extend your arms to starting position.

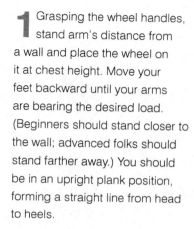

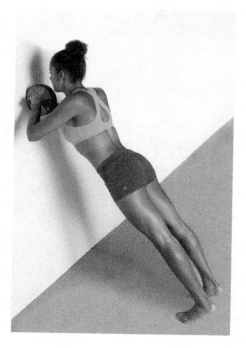

stork stand roll-up

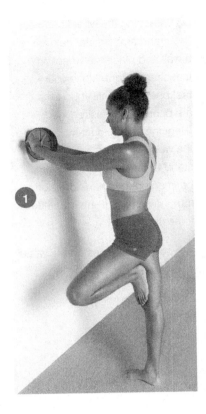

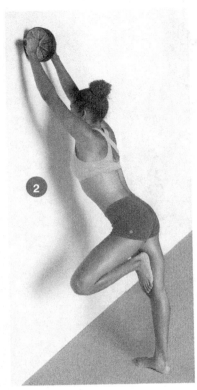

This is a suitable corrective exercise for fostering better core support and balance.

1 Grab the wheel handles with each hand and stand facing the wall. Place the wheel on the wall at chest height. Once in position, lift one foot off the ground however you feel comfortable.

2 Slowly roll the wheel up, only going as far as you can maintain proper neutral spine position. Hold.

Return to starting position and realign your posture.

child's pose

target: lower back

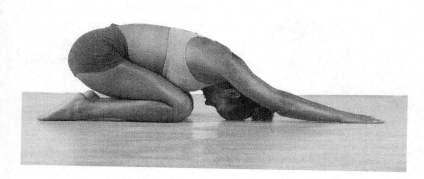

THE POSITION: Get on your hands and knees and rest your butt on your heels. Extend your arms forward and let your forehead rest on the floor, allowing your back to relax.

mad cat

target: lower back

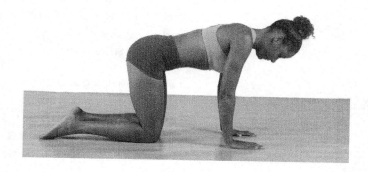

1 Get on your hands and knees.

2 Inhale and pull your belly button in, causing your back to round.

As you exhale, slowly relax your body to return to starting position.

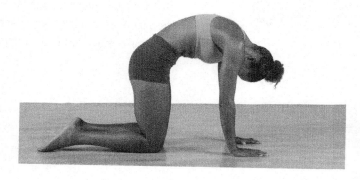

cobra

target: chest

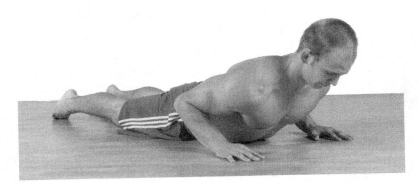

THE POSITION: Lie flat on your stomach with your legs extended behind you. Place your hands directly underneath your shoulders and press up lightly, allow your chest to open. Hold and then relax.

knee roll

target: torso, hips

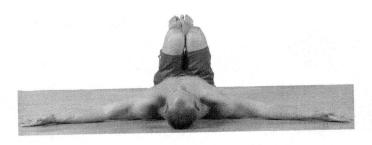

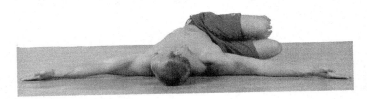

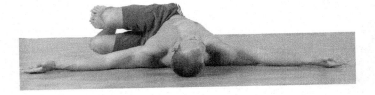

1 Lie with your knees bent and your feet flat on the floor. Place your arms straight out to your sides in a "T" position.

2 While inhaling through your nose, allow your knees to drop gently to the right without discomfort. Exhale and hold this position for a comfortable moment.

3 Inhale and bring your knees back to center, then gently drop them to your left. Exhale and hold this position for a comfortable moment.

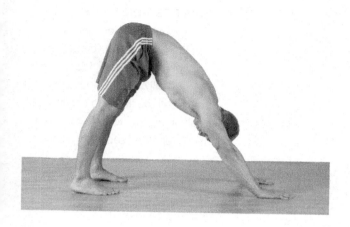

THE POSITION: From a plank position, push your hips back until your body forms an inverted "V." Make sure your fingers are spread wide and you're pressing into your whole hand. Press your heels toward the floor as you lift your tailbone up and back. Avoid forcing the move.

pelvic tilt

target: core

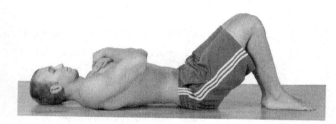

1 Lie on your back with your knees bent and feet on the floor.

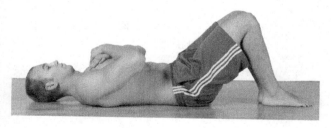

2 Contract your abdominals and slowly push the small of your back into the floor—pretend that you're trying to compress a sponge that's under the small of your back. Hold for 10 seconds.

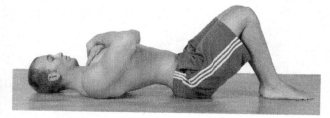

3 Now try to arch your lower back as much as is comfortable.

Release and allow the small of your back to return to neutral.

pelvic lift

target: abs, butt, lower back

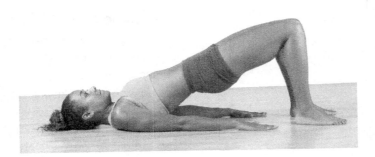

THE POSITION: Lie on your back with your knees bent and feet on the floor, resting your arms alongside your body. Press both feet equally into the floor to lift your pelvis off the floor. Do not lift your butt so high as to arch your back. Hold for 3 to 5 seconds.

windmill

target: shoulders

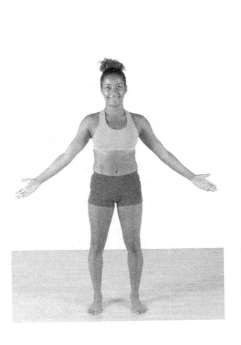
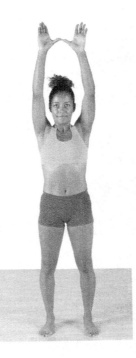

1 Stand with proper posture with your arms at your sides, palms facing forward.

2 Inhale deeply through your nose and slowly raise your arms out to the sides as high as is comfortable. Try to touch your thumbs.

Exhale and slowly lower your arms.

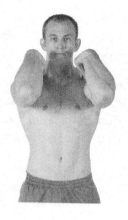 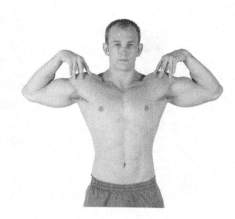

1 Stand with proper posture. Place your hands on your shoulders, elbows pointing forward. Slowly bring your elbows together in front of your body.

2 Bring your elbows back and squeeze your shoulder blades together. Hold for a moment, focusing on opening up your chest.

Return to starting position.

shoulder box

target: trapezius

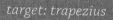

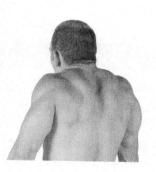 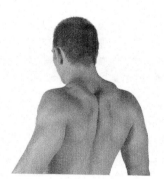

1 Stand with proper posture. Inhaling deeply through your nose, slowly lift up your shoulders.

2 Now pull your shoulders back and squeeze the shoulder blades together and down.

3 Exhaling through your lips, drop your shoulders and return to starting position.

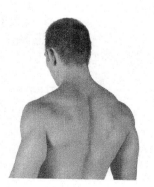

choker

target: shoulders, rotator cuff

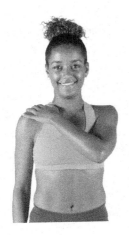
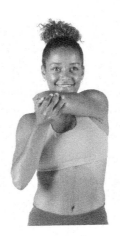

1 Stand with proper posture. Place your left hand on your right shoulder.

2 Place your right hand on your left elbow and gently press your left elbow toward your throat. Hold for a comfortable moment.

Switch sides and repeat.

lying knee to chest

target: lower back, gluteus maximus

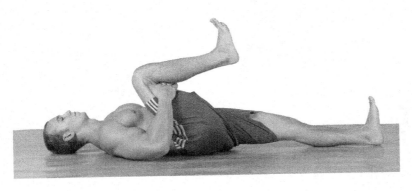

THE POSITION: Lie on the floor with your legs flat on the floor. Bring your right knee toward your chest and clasp both hands under your right thigh. Hold this position for a comfortable moment, feeling the stretch in the gluteal region.

Release the knee, switch sides and repeat.

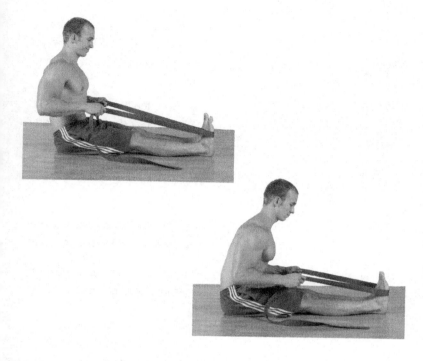

1 Sit on the floor with proper posture and extend both legs out in front of you. Loop a strap around the balls of both feet and hold the ends of the strap in each hand. Inhale deeply through your nose.

2 Now exhale through your lips and gently pull yourself forward by leading with your chest rather than rounding your back. Hold.

Switch sides and repeat.

rear calf stretch

target: calves

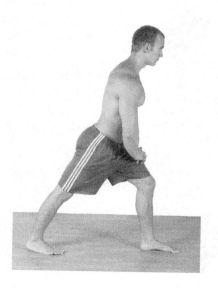

THE POSITION: Stand with proper posture. Keeping the heel down, slide your right leg as far back as you can. Bend your left knee until the desired stretch is felt in the calf area. Hold this stretch for a comfortable moment.

Switch sides and repeat.

gas pedal

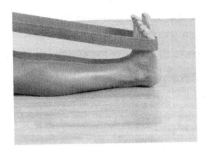
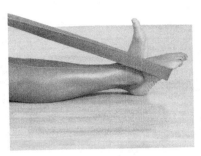

Caution: Do not force your toes in either direction. Be aware that your calf may cramp when extending your toes.

1 Sit on the floor with proper posture and extend both legs out in front of you. Loop a strap around the ball of one foot. Point your toes up and hold for several seconds.

2 Point your toes away from you and hold for several seconds.

Repeat a comfortable number of times then switch sides.

twister

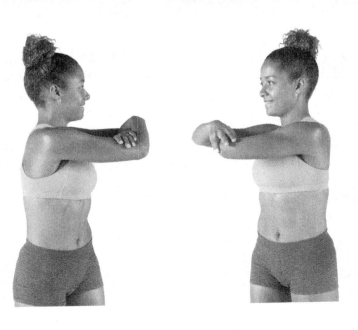

1 Stand with proper posture. Cross your arms in front of your chest and inhale slowly and deeply through your nose. While exhaling through your lips, slowly twist to your left. Hold the position for a comfortable moment and feel the stretch in your torso.

2 Inhale and return to the starting position before exhaling and twisting to your right. Hold the position for a comfortable moment and feel the stretch in your torso.

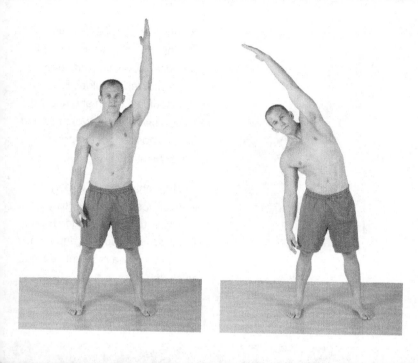

1 Stand with proper posture. Raise your left arm over your head to a comfortable height. Inhale deeply through your nose.

2 Now exhale through your lips and slowly and carefully lean to the right. Once you've leaned over enough to feel a gentle stretch along the right side of your body, hold this position for a comfortable moment.

Switch sides and repeat.

rock 'n' roll

target: lower back, torso

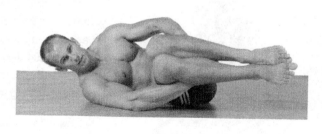

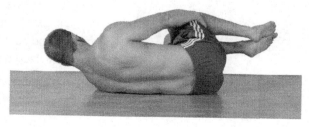

1–2 Lie on a mat and slowly bring both knees toward your chest. Gently reach around both legs and allow your shoulders to lift off the mat. While inhaling deeply through your nose and exhaling through your lips, slowly rock right and left, allowing your sides and shoulders to lift off the mat. Enjoy the relaxing feeling.

head tilt
target: neck

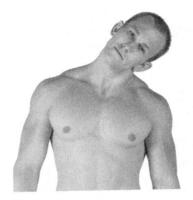 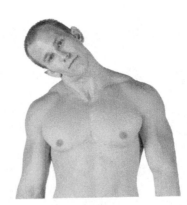

1 Stand with proper posture. While inhaling slowly through your nose, slowly tilt your head toward your left shoulder. Keep your shoulders down and relaxed. Exhale slowly through your lips and hold this position for a moment, feeling the stretch.

2 Now inhale slowly through your nose and slowly tilt your head to your right shoulder. Exhale slowly through your lips and hold this position for a moment, feeling the stretch.

tennis watcher
target: neck

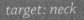

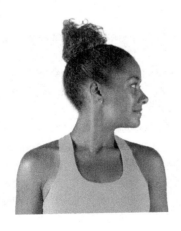 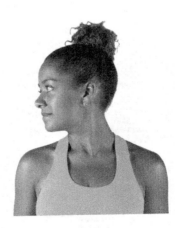

1 Stand with proper posture. While inhaling slowly through your nose, look to your left as far as you can without feeling discomfort. Exhale slowly through your lips and hold this position for a moment, feeling the stretch.

2 Now inhale slowly through your nose and look slowly to the right. Exhale slowly through your lips and hold this position for a moment, feeling the stretch.

index

other karl knopf books

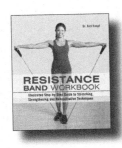

Resistance Band Workbook
$14.95
The ultimate tool for targeting, developing and healing every major muscle group, the resistance band is inexpensive, effective and portable. This book provides the most helpful workouts for noticeable results.

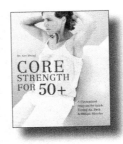

Core Strength for 50+
$15.95
Core Strength for 50+ provides the exercise and workout schedules that show anyone how to build and maintain strong muscles in the abs, obliques, lower back, butt and hips.

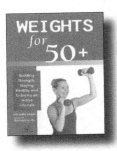

Weights for 50+
$14.95
Weight training is one of the most effective ways to get healthy and fight the physical signs of aging. *Weights for 50+* shows how easy it is for anyone to get started with weights.

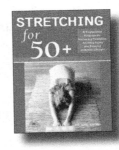

Stretching for 50+
$14.95
Based on the belief that individuals over 50 can do most of the same things as 20- and 30-year-olds, this book shows how to maintain and improve flexibility by incorporating stretching into one's life.

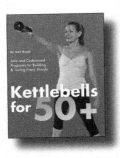

Kettlebells for 50+
$14.95
Offers progressive programs that will improve strength, foster core stability, increase hand-eye coordination, boost mind-body awareness, and enhance sports performance.

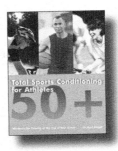

Total Sports Conditioning for Athletes 50+
$14.95
Provides sport-specific workouts that allow aging athletes to maintain the flexibility, strength, and speed needed to win.

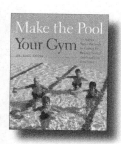

Make the Pool Your Gym
$14.95
Shows how to create an effective and efficient water workout that can build strength, improve cardiovascular fitness and burn calories.

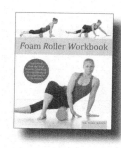

Foam Roller Workbook
$14.95
Details a comprehensive program for using the foam roller to recover from injury, reverse everyday pain and stay healthy in the future.

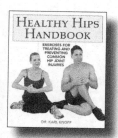

Healthy Hips Handbook
$14.95
Healthy Hips Handbook is designed to help prevent hip problems for some and, for those with existing hip problems, provide post-rehabilitation exercises.

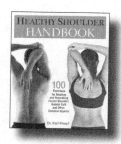

Healthy Shoulder Handbook
$15.95
Includes an overview of shoulder anatomy so anyone can use this friendly manual to strengthen an injured shoulder, identify the onset of a shoulder problem or better understand injury prevention.

To order these books call 800-377-2542 or 510-601-8301, fax 510-601-8307, e-mail ulysses@ulyssespress.com, or write to Ulysses Press, P.O. Box 3440, Berkeley, CA 94703. All retail orders are shipped free of charge. California residents must include sales tax. Allow two to three weeks for delivery.

acknowledgments

A special thanks goes to the whole Ulysses Press team, from Katherine Furman for her creative book concepts to Lily Chou who is able to translate my thoughts into a seamless flow of words. Also thanks goes to Claire Chun for her behind-the-screen work, as well as the excellent work of the photographic team of Rapt Productions and fitness skill set of models Bryan Johnson and Lache Kamani. Lastly to my wife of 35 years, Margaret, for allowing the time and space to work on this project.

about the author

KARL KNOPF is the author of many fitness handbooks including *Resistance Band Training, Core Strength for 50+, Kettlebells for 50+, Foam Roller Workbook, Healthy Shoulder Handbook* and *Make the Pool Your Gym.* He has also penned several textbooks on adaptive fitness. Dr. Karl (as his students fondly call him) has been involved with the health and fitness of the disabled and older adults for nearly four decades. He has served as a consultant on National Institutes of Health grants, as advisor to the PBS exercise series *Sit and Be Fit* and to the State of California on disabilities issues. Dr. Knopf, a frequent guest on radio and speaker at conferences, has been featured in the *Wall Street Journal* and is often quoted in magazines and newspapers. Dr. Knopf coordinates the Fitness Therapist Program at Foothill College and is the director of senior fitness at the International Sports Sciences Association (ISSA).

CPSIA information can be obtained
at www.ICGtesting.com
Printed in the USA
LVOW03s1812271115

464167LV00004B/9/P